VIETNAMESE
COOKBOOK

70 Easy Recipes For Pho Spring Rolls And Traditional Dishes From Vietnam

Contents

INTRODUCTION

CHAPTER 1: THE WORLD OF VIETNAMESE BREAKFAST RECIPES

CHAPTER 2: THE WORLD OF VIETNAMESE LUNCH RECIPES

CHAPTER 3: THE WORLD OF VIETNAMESE DINNER RECIPES

CHAPTER 4: THE WORLD OF VIETNAMESE DESSERT RECIPES

CHAPTER 5: THE WORLD OF VIETNAMESE SNACK RECIPES

CONCLUSION

Introduction

The rebirth of Vietnam as a tourist location has had a major effect in the country over the past years. However, one of the great results is that there are many individuals now who are finding out more about the Vietnamese cooking. These dishes are broadly viewed as among the best dishes on the planet and each dish is generally prepared with a range of flavors and spices.

Every locale of Vietnam has new flavored dishes alongside the traditional dishes of these locales. Street food is served everywhere as you travel anywhere in Vietnam. Grabbing a plastic stool and a street snack at a side of the road is perhaps one of the most ideal approaches to encounter Vietnamese food and communicate with the local people.

In this book, you will learn various recipes originated from Vietnam. This book contains 70 recipes that are traditionally cooked in Vietnam. The recipe section will include breakfast, lunch, dinner, snacks, and sweet dishes. All these recipes are detailed with easy to follow instructions and detailed ingredients that help you out in cooking by yourself at home. So, start reading this amazing book now!

Chapter 1: The World of Vietnamese Breakfast Recipes

There are many traditional dishes that are eaten as the morning meal in Vietnam. Following are traditional breakfast recipes that are loved by Vietnamese people around the world:

1.1 Vietnamese Bread Recipe

Preparation Time: 30 minutes
Cooking Time: 30 minutes
Serving: 4

Ingredients:

- Instant yeast, one packet
- Bread flour, one pound
- Sugar, three tablespoon
- Unsalted butter, two tablespoon
- Water, one cup (room temperature)
- Kosher salt, one teaspoon

Instructions:

1. Take a large bowl.
2. Add the instant yeast, sugar and water into the bowl.
3. Let the yeast dissolve for about five minutes.
4. Take another bowl and add the flour and salt into the bowl.
5. Make a round in the middle of the flour and add the yeast water into the round.
6. Mix the ingredients to form a dough.
7. Add the butter on the dough and knead it properly to get a soft dough.
8. Add the bread dough in a greased baking dish.
9. Bake the bread for twenty-five to thirty minutes.
10. The dish is ready to be served.

1.2 Vietnamese Rice Vermicelli Recipe

Preparation Time: 20 minutes
Cooking Time: 20 minutes
Serving: 4

Ingredients:

- Crushed peanuts, a quarter cup
- Chopped daikon radish, a quarter cup
- Chopped cilantro, three tablespoon
- Chopped English cucumber, one
- Chopped pickled carrots, a quarter cup
- Chopped fresh mint, three tablespoon
- Chopped fresh basil, three tablespoon
- Canola oil, one teaspoon
- Chopped shallots, two tablespoon
- Salt and pepper, to taste
- Shrimps, half pound
- Rice vermicelli noodles, one package
- Bean sprouts, one cup
- Chopped lettuce, one cup
- White vinegar, a quarter cup
- White sugar, two tablespoon
- Lime juice, two tablespoon
- Red pepper flakes, a quarter teaspoon
- Fish sauce, a quarter cup
- Chopped garlic, one teaspoon

Instructions:
1. Take a large bowl.
2. Add the white vinegar, fish sauce, chopped garlic, red pepper flakes, lime juice and white sugar.
3. Mix all the ingredients together and keep aside.
4. Add the oil into a large pan.
5. Add the chopped shallots into the pan and cook for about two to three minutes.
6. Add the shrimps into the pan and cook.
7. In the meantime, boil the rice noodles in a saucepan.

8. Drain the noodles when they are done.
9. Add the noodles, prepared sauce and rest of the ingredients into the pan.
10. Cook all the ingredients well.
11. The dish is ready to be served.

1.3 Vietnamese Mien Recipe

Preparation Time: 30 minutes
Cooking Time: 30 minutes
Serving: 4

Ingredients:

- Free range chicken, two pounds
- Glass noodles, one pack
- Chicken broth, four cups
- Garlic powder, one tablespoon
- Chopped cilantro, one cup
- Sliced red onion, one cup
- Canola oil, two tablespoon
- Chopped green onions, for garnishing
- Fried shallots, one cup

Instructions:
1. Take a large saucepan.
2. Add the canola oil and sliced red onions into the pan.
3. Cook the onions well.
4. Add the broth and glass noodles.
5. Cook the glass noodles and then add the rest of the ingredients into the saucepan.
6. Cook the ingredients for ten to fifteen minutes.
7. Your dish is ready to be served.

1.4 Vietnamese Rice Flour Crepes Recipe

Preparation Time: 10 minutes
Cooking Time: 15 minutes
Serving: 2

Ingredients:

- White sugar, one teaspoon
- Ground turmeric, a quarter teaspoon
- Coconut milk, one cup
- Rice flour, half cup
- Water, half cup
- Salt, half teaspoon

For filling:

- Minced shallots, two teaspoon
- Vegetable oil, two tablespoon
- Fresh shrimps, half cup
- Minced garlic, two teaspoon
- Bean sprouts, a quarter cup
- Fish sauce, two tablespoon
- Salt, to taste
- Black pepper, to taste

Instructions:

1. Mix all the ingredients for the crepes and set aside.
2. Take a large pan.
3. Heat it and add vegetable oil, shallots and garlic into the pan.
4. Cook the ingredients well and then add the bean sprouts and shrimps into the pan.
5. Cook for five minutes and then add the rest of the ingredients.
6. Dish out the shrimp mixture once it is cooked.
7. Add the crepes mixture on the pan and let it cook.
8. Add the shrimp mixture on top and fold the crepes.
9. Cook the crepes until they turn golden brown from both sides.
10. Your dish is ready to be served.

1.5 Vietnamese Breakfast Sandwich Recipe

Preparation Time: 10 minutes
Cooking Time: 20 minutes
Serving: 4

Ingredients:

- Fresh cilantro, half cup
- Pickled carrots and daikon, one cup
- Chopped chili pepper, one tablespoon
- Sliced cucumber, one
- Pork liver pate, two cups
- Soy sauce, two tablespoon
- Mayonnaise, three tablespoon
- Braised pork belly, one cup
- French baguette, as required
- Fried eggs, four

Instructions:

1. Cut the French baguette in half and toast the bread.
2. Add the mayonnaise and then the pork liver pate on one side of the baguette.
3. Layer the sandwich with braised pork belly, sliced cucumber, pickled carrot and daikon, and fresh cilantro.
4. Add the fried egg, soy sauce and chopped chili pepper on top.
5. Place the baguette slice on top.
6. Your dish is ready to be served.

1.6 Vietnamese Sticky Rice Recipe

Preparation Time: 20 minutes
Cooking Time: 20 minutes
Serving: 4

Ingredients:

- Glutinous rice, one cup
- Boneless chicken, one pound
- Salt, as required

- Cilantro as required
- Black pepper, to taste
- Chicken bouillon powder, two tablespoon
- Chinese sausages, half cup
- Roasted peanuts, half cup
- Fried onions, one cup
- Soy sauce, a quarter cup
- Water, one cup
- Spring onion oil, two tablespoon

Instructions:
1. Soak the glutinous rice in water for about half hour.
2. Take a large pan.
3. Add the spring onion oil into the pan and heat it.
4. Add the chicken and sausages into the oil.
5. Cook the ingredients well and then add the chicken bouillon powder, fried onion, salt and pepper into the pan.
6. Mix all the ingredients well and then add the rice along with the water.
7. Mix the ingredients well and then place a lid on top for about five minutes.
8. Add the rest of the ingredients and cook the dish for five to ten minutes.
9. Your dish is ready to be served.

1.7 Vietnamese Breakfast Fried Flour Cake Recipe

Preparation Time: 2 hours
Cooking Time: 10 minutes
Serving: 4

Ingredients:

- Salt, to taste
- Pepper, to taste
- Chicken bouillon powder, one teaspoon
- Dark soy sauce, two tablespoon
- Starch, one teaspoon
- Rice flour, two cups
- Water, four cup
- Oil, one teaspoon
- Oyster sauce, one teaspoon
- Light soy sauce, two teaspoon
- Vinegar, one teaspoon
- Sugar, two teaspoon

Instructions:

1. Take a large bowl.
2. Add the flour, water, starch, chicken bouillon powder, salt, pepper, and dark soy sauce into the bowl.
3. Mix all the ingredients well and fry the cake in a frying pan.
4. Mix the rest of the ingredients in a bowl.
5. Dish out the cake when it turns golden brown.
6. Pour the prepared sauce on top of the cake.
7. Your dish is ready to be served.

1.8 Vietnamese Quang Noodles Recipe

Preparation Time: 20 minutes
Cooking Time: 20 minutes
Serving: 4

Ingredients:

- Crushed peanuts, a quarter cup
- Chopped daikon radish, a quarter cup
- Chopped cilantro, three tablespoon
- Chopped English cucumber, one
- Chopped pickled carrots, a quarter cup
- Chopped fresh mint, three tablespoon
- Chopped fresh basil, three tablespoon
- Canola oil, one teaspoon
- Chopped shallots, two tablespoon
- Salt and pepper, to taste
- Chicken strips, half pound
- Rice noodles, one package
- Bean sprouts, one cup
- Chopped lettuce, one cup
- White vinegar, a quarter cup
- White sugar, two tablespoon
- Lime juice, two tablespoon
- Red pepper flakes, a quarter teaspoon
- Fish sauce, a quarter cup
- Chopped garlic, one teaspoon

Instructions:
1. Take a large bowl.
2. Add the white vinegar, fish sauce, chopped garlic, red pepper flakes, lime juice and white sugar.
3. Mix all the ingredients together and keep aside.
4. Add the oil into a large pan.
5. Add the chopped shallots into the pan and cook for about two to three minutes.
6. Add the chicken strips into the pan and cook.
7. In the meantime, boil the rice noodles in a saucepan.

8. Drain the noodles when they are done.
9. Add the noodles, prepared sauce and rest of the ingredients into the pan.
10. Cook all the ingredients well.
11. The dish is ready to be served.

1.9 Vietnamese Vermicelli Soup Recipe

Preparation Time: 20 minutes
Cooking Time: 20 minutes
Serving: 4

Ingredients:

- Kaffir lime leaves, a quarter cup
- Chopped daikon radish, a quarter cup
- Chopped cilantro, three tablespoon
- Cardamom pods, three
- Chopped pickled carrots, a quarter cup
- Fish sauce, three tablespoon
- Rice wine, three tablespoon
- Canola oil, one teaspoon
- Chopped shallots, two tablespoon
- Salt and pepper, to taste
- Chicken, half pound
- Rice vermicelli noodles, one package
- White vinegar, a quarter cup
- White sugar, two tablespoon
- Lime juice, two tablespoon
- Red pepper flakes, a quarter teaspoon
- Water, ten cups
- Chopped garlic, one teaspoon

Instructions:
1. Take a large bowl.
2. Add the white vinegar, fish sauce, chopped garlic, red pepper flakes, lime juice and white sugar.
3. Mix all the ingredients together and keep aside.

4. Add the oil into a large pan.
5. Add the chopped shallots into the pan and cook for about two to three minutes.
6. Add the chicken into the pan and cook.
7. In the meantime, boil the rice vermicelli noodles in a saucepan.
8. Drain the noodles when they are done.
9. Add the noodles, prepared sauce and rest of the ingredients into the pan.
10. Take a large sauce pan and add the rest of the ingredients into the pan.
11. Let the mixture boil and then add the noodle mixture into the pan.
12. Cook all the ingredients well.
13. The dish is ready to be served.

1.10 Vietnamese Beef Soup Recipe

Preparation Time: 30 minutes
Cooking Time: 10 minutes
Serving: 4

Ingredients:

- Star anise, four
- Cinnamon stick, one
- Beef stock, eight cups
- Sliced onion, one
- Beef strips, one pound
- Sesame oil, two teaspoon
- Fish sauce, half cup
- Oyster sauce, half tablespoon
- Mixed spices, one tablespoon
- Rice noodles, half pound
- Salt, to taste
- Black pepper, to taste
- Chopped fresh chives, as required
- Ginger piece, one

Instructions:
1. Take a large pan.

2. Add the oil and let it heat up.
3. Add in the sliced onion.
4. Cook the onion until soft.
5. Add in the ginger.
6. Mix the onions and ginger for two minutes and add in the beef pieces.
7. Add the spices and let it cook.
8. Cook the mixture for ten minutes.
9. Add in the fish sauce, oyster sauce and beef stock.
10. Add the noodles and rest of the ingredients.
11. Let the soup cook for ten to fifteen minutes.
12. Add the fresh chopped chives on top.
13. Your dish is ready to be served.

1.11 Vietnamese Breakfast Viscera Stew Recipe

Preparation Time: 10 minutes
Cooking Time: 30 minutes
Serving: 4

Ingredients:

- Chopped white shallots, one cup
- Viscera meat, half pound
- Sliced mushrooms, half pound
- Fish sauce, two tablespoon
- Soy sauce, three tablespoon
- White wine, half cup
- Minced garlic, one teaspoon
- Salt, to taste
- Beef stock, four cups
- Black pepper, to taste
- Olive oil, two tablespoon

Instructions:

1. Take a large pan.
2. Add the chopped shallots and olive oil into the pan.
3. Add in the minced garlic when the shallots turn soft and translucent.
4. Add the viscera meat into the pan and cook it.
5. Add in all the rest of the ingredients and cook the ingredients until the viscera meat is cooked.
6. Add the salt and pepper.
7. Cook the stew for about ten to fifteen minutes.
8. The dish is ready to be served.

1.12 Vietnamese Grilled Pork Vermicelli Recipe

Preparation Time: 20 minutes
Cooking Time: 20 minutes
Serving: 4

Ingredients:

- Crushed peanuts, a quarter cup
- Chopped daikon radish, a quarter cup
- Chopped cilantro, three tablespoon
- Chopped English cucumber, one
- Chopped pickled carrots, a quarter cup
- Chopped fresh mint, three tablespoon
- Chopped fresh basil, three tablespoon
- Canola oil, one teaspoon
- Chopped shallots, two tablespoon
- Salt and pepper, to taste
- Grilled pork pieces, half pound
- Rice vermicelli noodles, one package
- Bean sprouts, one cup
- Chopped lettuce, one cup
- White vinegar, a quarter cup
- White sugar, two tablespoon
- Lime juice, two tablespoon
- Red pepper flakes, a quarter teaspoon
- Fish sauce, a quarter cup
- Chopped garlic, one teaspoon

Instructions:
1. Take a large bowl.
2. Add the white vinegar, fish sauce, chopped garlic, red pepper flakes, lime juice and white sugar.
3. Mix all the ingredients together and keep aside.
4. Add the oil into a large pan.
5. Add the chopped shallots into the pan and cook for about two to three minutes.
6. Add the grilled pork pieces into the pan and cook.
7. In the meantime, boil the rice noodles in a saucepan.
8. Drain the noodles when they are done.
9. Add the noodles, prepared sauce and rest of the ingredients into the pan.
10. Cook all the ingredients well.
11. The dish is ready to be served.

Chapter 2: The World of Vietnamese Lunch Recipes

Classic Vietnamese lunch recipes are extremely delicious and worth eating. Following are some classic Vietnamese recipes that are rich in healthy nutrients and you can easily make them with the detailed instructions list in each recipe:

2.1 Vietnamese Savory Crepes Recipe

Preparation Time: 10 minutes
Cooking Time: 15 minutes
Serving: 2

Ingredients:

- White sugar, one teaspoon
- Ground turmeric, a quarter teaspoon
- Coconut milk, one cup
- Rice flour, half cup
- Water, half cup
- Salt, half teaspoon

For filling
- Oyster sauce, two tablespoon
- Minced shallots, two teaspoon
- Vegetable oil, two tablespoon
- Chopped green onions, half cup
- Minced garlic, two teaspoon
- Bean sprouts, a quarter cup
- Fish sauce, two tablespoon
- Salt, to taste
- Black pepper, to taste

Instructions:
1. Mix all the ingredients for the crepes and set aside.
2. Take a large pan.

3. Heat it and add vegetable oil, shallots and garlic into the pan.
4. Cook the ingredients well and then add the bean sprouts and green onions into the pan.
5. Cook for five minutes and then add the rest of the ingredients.
6. Dish out the bean sprout mixture once it is cooked.
7. Add the crepes mixture on the pan and let it cook.
8. Add the cooked mixture on top and fold the crepes.
9. Cook the crepes until they turn golden brown from both sides.
10. Your dish is ready to be served.

2.2 Vietnamese Crab and Tomato Noodle Soup Recipes

Preparation Time: 20 minutes
Cooking Time: 20 minutes
Serving: 4

Ingredients:

- Kaffir lime leaves, a quarter cup
- Chopped daikon radish, a quarter cup
- Chopped cilantro, three tablespoon
- Cardamom pods, three
- Chopped tomatoes, a quarter cup
- Fish sauce, three tablespoon
- Rice wine, three tablespoon
- Canola oil, one teaspoon
- Chopped shallots, two tablespoon
- Salt and pepper, to taste
- Crab meat, half pound
- Glass noodles, one package
- White vinegar, a quarter cup
- White sugar, two tablespoon
- Tomato paste, half cup
- Lime juice, two tablespoon
- Red pepper flakes, a quarter teaspoon
- Water, ten cups
- Chopped garlic, one teaspoon

Instructions:

1. Take a large bowl.
2. Add the white vinegar, fish sauce, chopped garlic, red pepper flakes, lime juice and white sugar.
3. Mix all the ingredients together and keep aside.
4. Add the oil into a large pan.
5. Add the chopped shallots into the pan and cook for about two to three minutes.
6. Add the chopped tomatoes, tomato paste, and crab meat into the pan and cook.
7. In the meantime, boil the rice vermicelli noodles in a saucepan.
8. Drain the noodles when they are done.
9. Add the noodles, prepared sauce and rest of the ingredients into the pan.
10. Take a large sauce pan and add the rest of the ingredients into the pan.
11. Let the mixture boil and then add the noodle mixture into the pan.
12. Cook all the ingredients well.
13. The dish is ready to be served.

2.3 Vietnamese Fried Spring Roll Recipe

Preparation Time: 10 minutes
Cooking Time: 30 minutes
Serving: 2

Ingredients:

- Rice paper rolls, half pound
- Minced garlic, one teaspoon
- Minced ginger, a quarter teaspoon
- Egg white, one
- Dried mushrooms, half cup
- Fish sauce, one tablespoon
- Sugar, three tablespoon
- Black pepper, as required
- Cilantro, half cup
- Salt, a quarter teaspoon
- Ground pork, one pound

- Soy sauce, as required
- Mung bean noodles, half cup
- Vegetable oil, for frying
- Ground white pepper, half teaspoon

Instructions:
1. Take a large pan.
2. Add a little bit oil and then the shallots, garlic and ginger into the pan.
3. Cook the ingredients well and then add the pork, mung bean noodles, carrots and rest of the ingredients.
4. Cook the ingredients well for about ten minutes.
5. Cook the mixture.
6. Add a tablespoon of the cooked mixture on the rice paper rolls and fold the rolls with the help of egg white.
7. Fry the rolls in a pan full of oil.
8. Dish out the rolls when they turn golden brown in color.
9. Your dish is ready to be served.

2.4 Vietnamese Caramelized Pork Rolls with Peanut Dipping Sauce Recipe

Preparation Time: 10 minutes
Cooking Time: 20 minutes
Serving: 2

Ingredients:

- Pork tenderloin, one pound
- Granulated sugar, half cup
- Salt to taste
- Black pepper to taste
- Fish sauce, two tablespoon
- Onion diced, one cup
- Sesame oil, one tablespoon
- Rice paper, one pack
- Chopped carrots, half cup
- Cucumber slices, half cup
- Cooked vermicelli, one cup

For the dipping sauce:
- Lemon juice, half cup
- Hoisin sauce, three tablespoon
- Chopped peanuts, half cup
- Minced garlic, one teaspoon
- Peanut oil, two tablespoon
- Salt, to taste
- Black pepper, to taste

Instructions:
1. Add the sesame oil into a pan.
2. Heat the oil well.
3. Add the pork tenderloins in the oil.
4. Cook the pork tenderloins well until they turn soft.
5. Add the fish sauce, granulated sugar, fish sauce, salt and black pepper.

6. Cook them for five minutes.
7. Cook the mixture again and keep stirring.
8. Add cooked pork on the rice paper and add the rest of the ingredients on top of the pork.
9. Fold roll and wrap it up.
10. Add the dipping sauce ingredients in a bowl and mix everything properly.
11. Pour the sauce on the roll.
12. Your dish is ready to be served.

2.5 Vietnamese Shrimp Soup Recipe

Preparation Time: 30 minutes
Cooking Time: 10 minutes
Serving: 4

Ingredients:

- Start anise, four
- Cinnamon stick, one
- Fish stock, eight cups
- Sliced onion, one
- Shrimp pieces, one pound
- Sesame oil, two teaspoon
- Fish sauce, half cup
- Oyster sauce, half tablespoon
- Mixed spices, one tablespoon
- Rice noodles, half pound
- Salt, to taste
- Black pepper, to taste
- Chopped fresh chives, as required
- Ginger piece, one

Instructions:
1. Take a large pan.
2. Add the oil and let it heat up.
3. Add in the sliced onion.
4. Cook the onion until soft.

5. Add in the ginger.
6. Mix the onions and ginger for two minutes and add in the shrimp pieces.
7. Add the spices and let it cook.
8. Cook the mixture for ten minutes.
9. Add in the fish sauce and the oyster sauce and fish stock.
10. Add the noodles and rest of the ingredients.
11. Let the soup cook for ten to fifteen minutes.
12. Add the fresh chopped chives on top.
13. Your dish is ready to be served.

2.6 Vietnamese Crispy Pork and Rice Noodles Recipe

Preparation Time: 30 minutes
Cooking Time: 10 minutes
Serving: 4

Ingredients:

- Butter, one tablespoon
- Cilantro, one cup
- Fresh ginger, one teaspoon
- Fish sauce, one tablespoon
- Soy sauce, one tablespoon
- Oyster sauce, half teaspoon
- Chili garlic sauce, two tablespoon
- Fresh cilantro leaves, half cup
- Crispy pork pieces, one pound
- Fresh basil leaves, a quarter cup
- Vegetable broth, one cup
- Rice noodles, as required

Instructions:

1. Add the fish sauce, soy sauce, oyster sauce and crispy pork pieces into a wok.
2. Cook the ingredients.
3. Add the noodles into the mixture once the sauce is ready.
4. Mix the noodles well and cook it for five minutes.
5. Add the rest of the ingredients into the wok.
6. Garnish the dish with chopped cilantro.
7. Your dish is ready to be served.

2.7 Vietnamese Stuffed Mushrooms Recipe

Preparation Time: 10 minutes

Cooking Time: 20 minutes
Serving: 4

Ingredients:

- Minced shrimp, one pound
- Mushrooms, half pound
- Lime juice, half cup
- Soy sauce, a quarter cup
- Oyster sauce, a quarter cup
- Fish sauce, a quarter cup
- Mozzarella cheese, one cup
- Chopped tomatoes, two
- Chopped red onion, one cup
- Chopped cilantro, half cup
- Chopped chives, half cup
- Vegetable oil, two tablespoon
- Salt, to taste
- Black pepper, to taste

Instructions:

1. Take a large pan.
2. Add the vegetable oil and minced shrimps into the pan.
3. Add the fish sauce, oyster sauce and soy sauce into the pan.
4. Add the rest of the spices, lime juice and tomatoes into the pan.
5. Wash the mushrooms and clean it from the middle.
6. Mix the rest of the ingredients in a bowl and add the cooked mixture into it.
7. Fill the mushrooms with the prepared mixture and then bake the mushrooms for ten minutes.
8. Your dish is ready to be served.

2.8 Vietnamese Grilled Pork with Scallions Recipe

Preparation Time: 30 minutes
Cooking Time: 10 minutes
Serving: 4

Ingredients:

- Cilantro, half cup
- Olive oil, two tablespoon
- Chopped tomatoes, one cup
- Lemon juice, half cup
- Mix spice powder, one tablespoon
- Salt, to taste
- Black pepper, to taste
- Fish sauce, one teaspoon
- Onion, one cup
- Pork pieces, one cup
- Chopped scallions, half cup
- Oyster sauce, half teaspoon
- Minced garlic, two tablespoon

Instructions:
1. Take a pan.
2. Add in the oil and onions.
3. Cook the onions until they become soft and fragrant.
4. Add in the chopped garlic.
5. Cook the mixture and add the tomatoes into it.
6. Add the spices and sauces.
7. Add the pork pieces into the pan.
8. Cook the dish five minutes.
9. Add the rest of the ingredients except cilantro and mix well.
10. Garnish the dish with chopped cilantro leaves.
11. Your dish is ready to be served.

2.9 Vietnamese Herb Salad Recipe

Preparation Time: 10 minutes
Cooking Time: 20 minutes
Serving: 4

Ingredients:

- Vietnamese salad dressing, two cups
- Minced ginger, two tablespoon
- Lemon juice, half cup
- Cilantro, one cup
- Olive oil, two tablespoon
- Chopped tomatoes, one cup
- Mixed fresh herbs, one cup
- Turmeric powder, one teaspoon
- Chopped onion, one cup
- Chopped lettuce leaves, one cup
- Soy sauce, half teaspoon
- Chopped avocado, one cup
- Minced garlic, two tablespoon

Instructions:
1. Take a large bowl.
2. Add the soy sauces and herbs in it.
3. Mix all the ingredients together.
4. Add the rest of the ingredients except the dressing and cilantro into the bowl and mix well.
5. Add the Vietnamese salad dressing on top of the salad.
6. Garnish the salad with the chopped cilantro.
7. Your dish is ready to be served.

2.10 Vietnamese Boiled Pork with Sour Shrimp Sauce Recipe

Preparation Time: 30 minutes
Cooking Time: 10 minutes
Serving: 4

Ingredients:

- Boiled pork, one pound
- Cilantro, half cup
- Sesame oil, two tablespoon
- Chopped tomatoes, one cup

- Shrimp paste, one cup
- Powdered cumin, one tablespoon
- Salt, to taste
- Black pepper, to taste
- Lemongrass, one teaspoon
- Chinese paprika, half teaspoon
- Diced kangkung, one cup
- Tamarind paste, half cup
- Minced garlic, two tablespoon
- Minced ginger, two tablespoon

Instructions:

1. Take a pan.
2. Add in the oil and onions.
3. Cook the onions until they become soft and fragrant.
4. Add in the chopped garlic and ginger.
5. Cook the mixture and add the tomatoes into it.
6. Add the spices.
7. Add the kangkung and shrimp paste into it.
8. Cook for five minutes.
9. Add in the boiled pork, lemongrass and tamarind paste.
10. Mix the ingredients carefully and cover the pan.
11. Garnish the dish with chopped cilantro leaves
12. Your dish is ready to be served.

2.11 Vietnamese Stir-Fried Baby Clams Recipe

Preparation Time: 30 minutes
Cooking Time: 10 minutes
Serving: 4

Ingredients:

- Fish broth, one cup
- Honey, one teaspoon
- Onion, one cup
- Brown sugar, two tablespoon
- Smoked paprika, half teaspoon
- Water, one cup
- Baby clams, two cups
- Mixed spices, two tablespoon
- Minced garlic, two tablespoon
- Minced ginger, two tablespoon
- Cilantro, half cup
- Olive oil, two tablespoon
- Chopped tomatoes, one cup

Instructions:
1. Take a pan.
2. Add in the oil and onions.
3. Cook the onions until they become soft and fragrant.
4. Add in the chopped garlic and ginger.
5. Cook the mixture and add the tomatoes into it.
6. Add the spices, honey, sugar and sauces.
7. Add the baby clams into it.
8. Cook for five minutes.
9. Garnish the dish with chopped cilantro leaves
10. Your dish is ready to be served.

2.12 Vietnamese Savory Rice Cake Recipe

Preparation Time: 2 hours
Cooking Time: 10 minutes
Serving: 4

Ingredients:

- Salt, to taste
- Black pepper, to taste
- Dark soy sauce, two tablespoon
- Starch, one teaspoon
- Rice flour, two cups
- Water, four cup

For the sauce:
- Cooked shrimps, one pound
- Nuoc mam cham, one cup
- Oil, one teaspoon
- Oyster sauce, one teaspoon
- Light soy sauce, two teaspoon
- Vinegar, one teaspoon
- Sugar, two teaspoon
- Chopped pickled radish, three tablespoon

Instructions:
1. Take a large bowl.
2. Add the flour, water, starch, salt, pepper, and dark soy sauce into the bowl.
3. Mix all the ingredients well and fry the cake in a frying pan.
4. Mix the rest of the ingredients for the sauce in a bowl.
5. Dish out the cake when it turns golden brown.
6. Pour the prepared shrimp sauce on top of the cake.
7. Your dish is ready to be served.

2.13 Vietnamese Meat Buns Recipe

Preparation Time: 30 minutes
Cooking Time: 25 minutes
Serving: 4

Ingredients:

- All-purpose flour, four cups
- Sesame seeds, as required
- Oyster sauce, half teaspoon
- Soy sauce, one teaspoon
- Milk, one cup
- Active yeast, half teaspoon
- Eggs, three
- Sugar, half cup
- Cooked pork meat, a quarter cup

Instructions:

1. In a large bowl, add the active yeast and sugar.
2. In a separate bowl, add in the dry ingredients.
3. Add the active yeast mixture into the dry ingredients.
4. Add the eggs.
5. Knead the dough.
6. Make small buns and place them on a baking tray.
7. Add the rest of the ingredients in a small bowl.
8. Add this mixture in between the buns and place it on the tray.
9. Brush the egg mixture on top.
10. Bake the buns for fifteen to twenty minutes.
11. The dish is ready to be served.

2.14 Vietnamese Grilled Beef with Pickled Vegetables Recipe

Preparation Time: 10 minutes
Cooking Time: 20 minutes
Serving: 2

Ingredients:

- Coconut aminos, three tablespoon
- Raw honey, two teaspoon
- Avocado oil, two tablespoon
- Minced garlic, two tablespoon
- Lime juice, two tablespoon
- Salt, to taste
- Black pepper, to taste
- Cilantro, half cup
- Olive oil, two tablespoon
- Sirloin steak, two pound
- Pickled vegetables, as required

Instructions:

1. Take a large bowl.
2. Add the salt, black pepper, sirloin steak, lime juice, coconut aminos, raw honey, minced garlic and raw honey into the bowl.
3. Add the prepared sauce on top of the sirloin steak.
4. Heat the grilling pan.
5. Add the olive oil on the grilling pan and add the marinated sirloin steak on top.
6. Grill the steak on both sides and then slice it up in pieces.
7. Serve the pickled vegetables on the sides.
8. Your dish is ready to be served.

2.15 Vietnamese Stir-Fried Egg Noodles Recipe

Preparation Time: 30 minutes
Cooking Time: 20 minutes
Serving: 4

Ingredients:

- Salt, to taste
- Black pepper, to taste
- Boiled noodles, two cups
- Broccoli florets, one cup
- Oyster sauce, half teaspoon
- Vegetable oil, one tablespoon
- Baby corns, half cup
- Minced garlic, two tablespoon
- Minced ginger, two tablespoon
- Cilantro, half cup
- Shitake mushrooms, one cup
- Fish sauce, two tablespoon
- Granulated sugar, two tablespoon
- Chicken stock, half cup
- Chopped tomatoes, one cup

Instructions:
1. Take a large pan.
2. Add in the oil, ginger and garlic.
3. Add the tomatoes and mix well.
4. Add the fish sauce, granulated sugar, oyster sauce and soy sauce into the pan.
5. Add the vegetables and noodles.
6. Mix everything well and then add the rest of the ingredients.
7. Cook the ingredients for ten minutes.
8. Your dish is ready to be served.

Chapter 3: The World of Vietnamese Dinner Recipes

Vietnamese dinner recipes are extremely healthy and loved by people everywhere in the world. Following are some classic dinner recipes that are rich in healthy nutrients and you can easily make them with the detailed instructions list in each recipe:

3.1 Vietnamese Turmeric and Dill Fish with Rice Recipe

Preparation Time: 30 minutes
Cooking Time: 10 minutes
Serving: 4

Ingredients:

- Turmeric powder, one tablespoon
- Chopped dill, half cup
- Sesame oil, two tablespoon
- Chopped red pepper, one tablespoon
- Cooked rice, two cup
- Powdered cumin, one tablespoon
- Salt, to taste
- Black pepper, to taste
- Lemongrass, one teaspoon
- Chinese paprika, half teaspoon
- Fish, one pound
- Caster sugar, two teaspoon
- Fish sauce, two tablespoon
- Tamarind paste, half cup
- Minced garlic, two tablespoon
- Minced ginger, two tablespoon

Instructions:
1. Take a large bowl.

2. Add the chopped dill, chopped red pepper, black pepper, salt, lemongrass, powdered cumin, Chinese paprika, caster sugar, fish sauce, minced ginger, tamarind paste and turmeric powder into the bowl.
3. Add the fish into the bowl and cover the fish completely in the mixture.
4. Take a large frying pan.
5. Add the oil in the pan.
6. Add the marinated fish and fry it until it turns golden brown.
7. Garnish the fish with chopped cilantro and serve it with rice.
8. Your dish is ready to be served.

3.2 Vietnamese Beef and Green Papaya Salad Recipe

Preparation Time: 10 minutes
Cooking Time: 25 minutes
Serving: 4

Ingredients:

- Cooked beef cubes, one cup
- Carrot sliced, one cup
- Red bell pepper sliced, one cup
- Ginger, one tablespoon
- Garlic powder, two teaspoon
- Fish sauce, half teaspoon
- Sesame oil, one teaspoon
- Soy sauce, one teaspoon
- Sriracha, one tablespoon
- Lime juice, one tablespoon
- Green papaya pieces, one cup
- Salt, to taste
- Pepper, to taste

Instructions:
1. Take a large bowl and add beef cubes into it.
2. Add the ginger and garlic powder.
3. Mix well.
4. Add the green papaya slices, carrot slices and red bell pepper into it.
5. Add the salt and pepper as you like.

6. Add the sesame oil and mix well so that a consistent mixture is obtained.
7. Add the sriracha and rest of the ingredients into the mixture.
8. Mix all the ingredients.
9. Your salad is ready to be served.

3.3 Vietnamese Roasted Salmon Recipe

Preparation Time: 10 minutes
Cooking Time: 30 minutes
Serving: 2

Ingredients:

- Turmeric powder, one teaspoon
- Onion, one cup
- Salmon filet pieces, half pound
- Smoked paprika, half teaspoon
- Minced garlic, two tablespoon
- Minced ginger, two tablespoon
- Lemon juice, half cup
- Soy sauce, two tablespoon
- Oyster sauce, two teaspoon
- Fish sauce, two teaspoon
- Chinese paprika, one teaspoon
- Olive oil, two tablespoon
- Chopped tomatoes, one cup

Instructions:
1. Take a pan.
2. Add in the oil and onions.
3. Cook the onions until they become soft and fragrant.
4. Add in the chopped garlic and ginger.
5. Cook the mixture and add the tomatoes into it.
6. Add the spices and sauce.
7. Add the salmon pieces into it.
8. Mix the ingredients carefully and place the mixture into the oven.
9. Add cilantro on top.

10.   Drizzle any preferred sauce on top of the fish.
11.   Your dish is ready to be served.

3.4 Vietnamese Beef and Carrot Salad Recipe

Preparation Time: 10 minutes
Cooking Time: 25 minutes
Serving: 4

Ingredients:

- Cooked beef cubes, one cup
- Carrot sliced, one cup
- Ginger, one tablespoon
- Garlic powder, two teaspoon
- Fish sauce, half teaspoon
- Sesame oil, one teaspoon
- Soy sauce, one teaspoon
- Sriracha, one tablespoon
- Lime juice, one tablespoon
- Salt, to taste
- Pepper, to taste

Instructions:

1. Take a large bowl and add beef cubes into it.
2. Add the ginger and garlic powder.
3. Mix well.
4. Add the carrot slices into it.
5. Add the salt and pepper as you like.
6. Add the sesame oil and mix well so that a consistent mixture is obtained.
7. Add the sriracha and rest of the ingredients into the mixture.
8. Mix all the ingredients.
9. Your salad is ready to be served.

3.5 Vietnamese Lamb Shanks Recipe

Preparation Time: 30 minutes
Cooking Time: 10 minutes
Serving: 4

Ingredients:

- Cooked sweet potatoes, two cup
- Mix spice, one teaspoon
- Onion, one cup
- Smoked paprika, half teaspoon
- Chinese dried chilies, half cup
- Minced garlic, two tablespoon
- Minced ginger, two tablespoon
- Lemon juice, half cup
- Oyster sauce, half cup
- Lamb shanks, half pound
- Olive oil, two tablespoon
- Chopped tomatoes, one cup

Instructions:

1. Take a pan.
2. Add in the oil and onions.
3. Cook the onions until they become soft and fragrant.
4. Add in the chopped garlic and ginger.
5. Cook the mixture and add the tomatoes into it.
6. Add the spices.
7. Add the sweet potato and rest of the ingredients into it.
8. Mix the ingredients carefully.
9. Add cilantro on top.
10. Your dish is ready to be served.

3.6 Vietnamese Spicy Summer Rolls Recipe

Preparation Time: 10 minutes
Cooking Time: 20 minutes
Serving: 2

Ingredients:

- Beef pieces, one pound
- Granulated sugar, half cup
- Salt to taste
- Black pepper to taste
- Fish sauce, two tablespoon
- Onion diced, one cup
- Sesame oil, one tablespoon
- Rice paper, one pack
- Chopped carrots, half cup
- Cucumber slices, half cup
- Cooked vermicelli, one cup

For the hot sauce:

- Lemon juice, half cup
- Hoisin sauce, three tablespoon
- Chopped red chilies, half cup
- Minced garlic, one teaspoon
- Chili oil, two tablespoon
- Salt, to taste
- Black pepper, to taste

Instructions:

1. Add the sesame oil into a pan.
2. Heat the oil well.
3. Add the beef pieces in the oil.
4. Cook the beef pieces well until they turn soft.
5. Add the fish sauce, granulated sugar, fish sauce, salt and black pepper.
6. Cook them for five minutes.
7. Cook the mixture again and keep stirring.
8. Add cooked beef on the rice paper and add the rest of the ingredients on top of the beef.

9. Fold the roll and wrap it up.
10. Add the hot sauce ingredients in a bowl and mix everything properly.
11. Pour the sauce on the roll.
12. Your dish is ready to be served.

3.7 Vietnamese Beef and Lemongrass Salad Recipe

Preparation Time: 10 minutes
Cooking Time: 10 minutes
Serving: 2

Ingredients:

- Beef, half pound
- Lemongrass, two teaspoon
- Wine vinegar, one cup
- Caster sugar, a quarter teaspoon
- Spring onions, half cup
- Bean sprouts, two cups
- Sirarcha, half cup
- Pepper, as required
- Cilantro, half cup
- Salt, a quarter teaspoon
- Soy sauce, as required
- Bird's eye chili, half cup
- Salad dressing, half cup

Instructions:
1. Cook the beef by boiling it well.
2. Mix all the ingredients along with the bean sprouts and spring onions.
3. Add the salad dressing in a bowl and beat it well.
4. Drizzle the salad dressing on top of the salad mixture.
5. Your dish is ready to be served.

3.8 Vietnamese Pork Curry Recipe

Preparation Time: 30 minutes
Cooking Time: 10 minutes
Serving: 4

Ingredients:

- Brown sugar, one tablespoon
- Cilantro, half cup
- Sesame oil, two tablespoon
- Chopped tomatoes, one cup
- Pork, one cup
- Oyster sauce, one tablespoon
- Salt, to taste
- Black pepper, to taste
- Lemongrass, one teaspoon
- Chinese paprika, half teaspoon
- Minced garlic, two tablespoon
- Water, as needed
- Minced ginger, two tablespoon

Instructions:

1. Take a pan.
2. Add in the oil and onions.
3. Cook the onions until they become soft and fragrant.
4. Add in the chopped garlic and ginger.
5. Cook the mixture and add the tomatoes into it.
6. Add the spices.
7. Add the pork pieces into it.
8. Cook for five minutes.
9. Add in the brown sugar, lemongrass and some water.
10. Mix the ingredients carefully and cover the pan.
11. Garnish the dish with chopped cilantro leaves.
12. Your dish is ready to be served.

3.9 Vietnamese Veggie Curry Recipe

Preparation Time: 20 minutes
Cooking Time: 20 minutes
Serving: 4

Ingredients:

- Oyster sauce, one tablespoon
- Chinese chili peppers, two
- Fish sauce, one tablespoon
- Soy sauce, half tablespoon
- Minced garlic, two teaspoon
- Cooking oil, three tablespoon
- Hot sauce, half cup
- Mixed vegetables, two cups
- Salt, as required
- Chopped fresh cilantro, as required

Instructions:

1. Take a large pan.
2. Add the cooking oil into the pan and heat it.
3. Add the vegetables into the pan and stir-fry it.
4. Add the minced garlic into the pan.
5. Add the soy sauce, fish sauce, Chinese chili peppers, hot sauce and rest of the ingredients into the mixture.
6. Cook the dish for ten minutes and add some water for curry.
7. Dish out the vegetables and garnish them with chopped fresh cilantro leaves.
8. Your dish is ready to be served.

3.10 Vietnamese Prawn and Noodle Salad with Crispy Shallots Recipe

Preparation Time: 10 minutes
Cooking Time: 25 minutes
Serving: 4

Ingredients:

- Cooked prawns, one cup
- Ginger powder, one tablespoon
- Garlic powder, two teaspoon
- Fish sauce, half teaspoon
- Sesame oil, one teaspoon
- Soy sauce, one teaspoon
- Sriracha, one tablespoon
- Lime juice, one tablespoon
- Noodles, one pack
- Salt, to taste
- Pepper, to taste
- Shallots, half cup

Instructions:
1. Take a large bowl and add prawns into it.
2. Add the ginger and garlic powder.
3. Mix well.
4. Add the salt and pepper as per your taste.
5. Add the sesame oil and mix well so that a consistent mixture is obtained.
6. Add the noodles, prawns and the rest of the ingredients into the mixture.
7. Fry the shallots in oil until they turn crispy.
8. Add the shallots on top of the mixture.
9. Your salad is ready to be served.

3.11 Vietnamese Basil Chicken Recipe

Preparation Time: 30 minutes
Cooking Time: 10 minutes
Serving: 4

Ingredients:

- Basil leaves, half cup
- Chicken, one pound
- Sesame oil, two tablespoon
- Chopped tomatoes, one cup
- Lemon juice, one cup
- Fish sauce, one tablespoon
- Salt, to taste
- Black pepper, to taste
- Lemongrass, one teaspoon
- Onion, one cup
- Chicken broth, one cup
- Chinese paprika, half teaspoon
- Minced garlic, two tablespoon
- Minced ginger, two tablespoon

Instructions:

1. Take a pan.
2. Add in the oil and onions.
3. Cook the onions until they become soft and fragrant.
4. Add in the chopped garlic and ginger.
5. Cook the mixture and add the tomatoes into it.
6. Add the spices.
7. Add the chicken pieces into it.
8. Cook for five minutes.
9. Add in the lemongrass.
10. Add in the broth and lemon juice.
11. Mix the ingredients carefully and cover the pan.
12. Garnish the dish with chopped basil leaves.
13. Your dish is ready to be served.

3.12 Vietnamese Garlic Noodles Recipe

Preparation Time: 30 minutes
Cooking Time: 10 minutes
Serving: 4

Ingredients:

- Butter, one tablespoon
- Cilantro, one cup
- Fresh ginger, one teaspoon
- Fish sauce, one tablespoon
- Soy sauce, one tablespoon
- Oyster sauce, half teaspoon
- Chili garlic sauce, two tablespoon
- Fresh cilantro leaves, half cup
- Fresh basil leaves, a quarter cup
- Vegetable broth, one cup
- Garlic noodles, as required

Instructions:

1. Add the butter, ginger, fish sauce, soy sauce, oyster sauce, chili garlic sauce, basil leaves, and vegetable broth into a wok.
2. Cook the ingredients.
3. Add the noodles into the mixture once the sauce is ready.
4. Mix the noodles well and cook it for five minutes.
5. Add the cilantro into the dish.
6. Your dish is ready to be served.

3.13 Vietnamese Salmon with Roasted Cashew Rice Recipe

Preparation Time: 10 minutes
Cooking Time: 30 minutes
Serving: 2

Ingredients:

- Maple syrup, one teaspoon
- Cashew rice, one cup
- Salmon, half pound
- Ground ginger, a quarter teaspoon
- Spices, as you like
- Chopped red pepper, as required
- Cilantro, half cup
- Salt, a quarter teaspoon

Instructions:
1. Roast the cashew rice well in an oven for ten minutes.
2. In the meantime, add the maple syrup, ginger and red pepper in a bowl.
3. Marinate the salmon in the bowl.
4. Cook the salmon well in a pan adding all the spices and ingredients.
5. Serve the rice with salmon.
6. Your dish is ready to be served.

3.14 Vietnamese Fried Eggplant Soup Recipe

Preparation Time: 10 minutes
Cooking Time: 30 minutes
Serving: 4

Ingredients:

- Chopped white onions, one cup
- Fried eggplant, one cup
- Fresh chopped cilantro, half cup
- Unsalted butter, three tablespoon
- Oyster sauce, one teaspoon
- Minced garlic, one teaspoon
- Fish sauce, half teaspoon
- Vegetable stock, one cup
- Coconut milk, half cup
- Coconut cream, one cup

Instructions:

1. Take a large pan.
2. Add the chopped onions and butter in the pan.
3. Add in the minced garlic.
4. Add the fried eggplant in the pan.
5. Add in all the rest of the ingredients and cook the ingredients until they are done.
6. Blend the soup well.
7. Cook for an extra few minutes.
8. The dish is ready to be served.

3.15 Vietnamese Fried Pork Chops Recipe

Preparation Time: 30 minutes
Cooking Time: 10 minutes
Serving: 4

Ingredients:

- Cilantro, half cup
- Olive oil, two tablespoon
- Chopped tomatoes, one cup
- Lemon juice, half cup
- Mix spice powder, one tablespoon
- Salt, to taste
- Black pepper, to taste
- Fish sauce, one teaspoon
- Onion, one cup
- Pork chops, one cup
- Oyster sauce, half teaspoon
- Minced garlic, two tablespoon

Instructions:

1. Take a bowl.
2. Add in the oil and chopped onions.
3. Mix the onions well.
4. Add in the chopped garlic and pork chops.
5. Stir the mixture and add the tomatoes into it.
6. Add the spices and sauces.
7. Fry the pork chops until they become light brown in color.
8. Garnish the dish with chopped cilantro leaves.
9. Your dish is ready to be served.

3.16 Vietnamese Pork Soup Recipe

Preparation Time: 10 minutes
Cooking Time: 20 minutes

Serving: 4

Ingredients:

- Minced garlic, two tablespoon
- Minced ginger, two tablespoon
- Pork, one cup
- Cilantro, half cup
- Diced carrots, one cup
- Olive oil, two tablespoon
- Fish sauce, half cup
- Vegetable stock, half cup
- Chopped tomatoes, one cup
- Hot sauce, half cup
- Onion, one cup
- Bell peppers, one cup
- Water, one cup
- Oyster sauce, half teaspoon
- Soy sauce, one cup

Instructions:

1. Take a pan.
2. Add in the oil and onions.
3. Cook the onions until they become soft and fragrant.
4. Add in the chopped garlic and ginger.
5. Cook the mixture and add the tomatoes into it.
6. Add the sauces.
7. Add the pork into the pan.
8. Cook it well until becomes tender.
9. Mix the ingredients carefully and cover your pan.
10. Add the vegetables into the mixture.
11. Add the water and stock into the mixture and cover the pan.
12. Let the soup cook for ten to fifteen minutes straight.
13. Add the cilantro on top.
14. Your dish is ready to be served.

3.17 Vietnamese Spicy Beef Recipe

Preparation Time: 30 minutes
Cooking Time: 20 minutes
Serving: 4

Ingredients:

- Sesame oil, two tablespoon
- Sugar, one teaspoon
- Oyster sauce, two tablespoon
- Pepper to taste
- Salt, as required
- Chinese cooking wine, two teaspoon
- Soy sauce, two tablespoon
- Beef chunks, two pounds
- Vegetable oil, two tablespoon
- Japanese seven spices, as needed

Instructions:

1. Add the oil in a large pan.
2. Add in the beef and cook it properly.
3. Add the rest of the ingredients.
4. Add the Japanese seven spices and once the dish thickens switch off the heat.
5. Your dish is ready to be served.

3.18 Vietnamese Tomato and Pineapple Soup Recipe

Preparation Time: 30 minutes
Cooking Time: 20 minutes
Serving: 4

Ingredients:

- Diced pineapple, one cup
- Onion, one cup
- Oyster sauce, half teaspoon
- Water, one cup

- Minced garlic, two tablespoon
- Soy sauce, two tablespoon
- Chopped cilantro, half cup
- Olive oil, two tablespoon
- Water, one cup
- Vegetable stock, half cup
- Cherry tomatoes, one cup

Instructions:
1. Take a pan.
2. Add in the oil and onions.
3. Cook the onions until they become soft and fragrant.
4. Add in the chopped garlic.
5. Cook the mixture and add the cherry tomatoes into it.
6. Add the spices and sauces.
7. Add the diced pineapple into it.
8. Mix in the rest of the ingredients and cover the pan.
9. Let the soup cook for ten to fifteen minutes straight.
10. Add chopped cilantro on top.
11. Your dish is ready to be served.

Chapter 4: The World of Vietnamese Dessert Recipes

You should really try Vietnamese desserts if you have a sweet tooth. Following are some yummy dessert recipes that are rich in healthy nutrients:

4.1 Vietnamese Pandan Rice Cake Recipe

Preparation Time: 10 minutes
Cooking Time: 20 minutes
Serving: 4

Ingredients:

- Sweet pandan rice, two cup
- Salt, a pinch
- Bread flour, half cup
- Coconut milk, one cup
- Lime zest, half teaspoon
- Mung bean paste, one cup
- Baking powder, one teaspoon
- Vanilla essence, half teaspoon

Instructions:
1. Add the bread flour into a large bowl.
2. Cook the pandan rice in the rice cooking pan.
3. Add the rice into the bowl when they are cooked and mix them.
4. Add the lime zest into the bowl and mix well.
5. Add some water and boil the whole mixture for ten minutes.
6. Cool the mixture and then add the vanilla essence, baking powder and coconut milk into it.
7. Mix the ingredients well.
8. Add the batter into the cupcake molds.
9. Add the mung bean paste in the center of the mixture.
10. Bake the rice cake.
11. Dish out the cake when it is done.
12. Your dish is ready to be served.

4.2 Vietnamese Colored Jellies Recipe

Preparation Time: 40 minutes
Cooking Time: 10 minutes
Serving: 4

Ingredients:

- Fresh longans, one pound
- Coconut juice, one liter
- Agar powder, fifteen grams
- Rock sugar, two hundred grams
- Mint syrup, two teaspoon
- Strawberry syrup, two teaspoon
- Water, half liter
- Condensed milk, one cup

Instructions:
1. Peel the longans and remove seeds from them.
2. Grind the longans and set aside.
3. Take a bowl and add the rock sugar and jelly powder in it.
4. Add the coconut water into the bowl and mix well.
5. Heat the mixture so that all ingredients get dissolved.
6. Add the mint syrup and strawberry syrup in two separate bowls.
7. Add the clear agar jelly in both bowls.
8. Add the condensed milk in it and mix well.
9. Add the grinded longans and mix well.
10. Your colored jelly is ready to be served.

4.3 Vietnamese Coconut Dumplings Recipe

Preparation Time: 50 minutes
Cooking Time: 30 minutes
Serving: 4

Ingredients:

- Crushed coconut, five tablespoon
- Cinnamon powder, half tablespoon

- Sweet vinegar, one tablespoon
- Milk, one cup
- Vegetable oil, one tablespoon
- All-purpose flour, one cup
- Whole wheat flour, half cup
- Salt, to taste
- Water, to kneed

Instructions:

1. Take a bowl and add the flour into it.
2. Add lukewarm water in it.
3. Set aside for half hour.
4. Add the whole wheat flour into the bowl.
5. Add the salt and milk in it.
6. Combine the ingredients to form a soft dough.
7. Kneed it for ten minutes.
8. Take a small bowl.
9. Add the cinnamon powder, sweet vinegar and crushed coconut in the bowl.
10. Make round balls from the dough and add the coconut mixture in between.
11. Steam the dumplings for ten minutes.
12. Your dish is ready to be served.

4.4 Vietnamese Sesame Waffles Recipe

Preparation Time: 30 minutes
Cooking Time: 10 minutes
Serving: 4

Ingredients:

- Rice flour, one cup
- Eggs, two
- Chopped fresh cilantro, half cup
- Coconut milk, one cup
- Salt to taste
- Sesame oil, one teaspoon
- Sesame seeds, half cup

Instructions:

1. Heat the waffle maker.
2. Beat the egg yolks in a separate bowl.
3. Add the egg yolks in the egg whites and delicately mix them with a spatula.
4. Combine the eggs and the rest of the ingredients.
5. Pour the mixture into the waffle maker.
6. Close the waffle maker.
7. Let the waffle cook for five to six minutes approximately.
8. Add on top of the waffles the sesame seeds.
9. Your dish is ready to be served.

4.5 Vietnamese Traditional Yellow Dessert Recipe

Preparation Time: 10 minutes
Cooking Time: 20 minutes
Serving: 4

Ingredients:

- Yellow color, three drops
- Rice, one cup
- Baking powder, four teaspoon
- Coconut milk, one cup
- All-purpose flour, one and a half cup
- Baking soda, one teaspoon
- Eggs, two
- Brown sugar, one cup
- Tapioca starch, one tablespoon
- Salt, to taste

Instructions:
1. Take a large bowl and add the eggs into it.
2. Beat the eggs until they turn frothy.
3. Add the baking powder and coconut milk into it.
4. Add the brown sugar and beat the mixture for five minutes.
5. Add all the dried ingredients in a separate bowl.
6. Mix them thoroughly.
7. Cook the mixture until it turns thick.
8. Cook the rice in rice cooking pan.
9. Add the yellow color to the rice.
10. Add the rice into the cooked mixture.

11.   Your dish is ready to be served.

4.6 Vietnamese Dessert Soup with Mung Beans Recipe

Preparation Time: 10 minutes
Cooking Time: 20 minutes
Serving: 4

Ingredients:

- Mung beans, half cup
- Banana slices, one cup
- Plain yogurt, half cup
- Milk, half cup
- Sugar, half cup
- Apples, half cup
- Melon, half cup
- Mixed fruit juice, half cup
- Ice cubes, as required

Instructions:
1. Take a blender and add the milk into it.
2. Add the mung beans in it.
3. Add the banana slices into it.
4. Blend it for few minutes.
5. Add the plain yogurt into it.
6. Add the fruit juice into it.
7. Add the melon, sugar and apples into it.
8. Your dish is ready to be served.

4.7 Vietnamese Coconut Pudding Recipe

Preparation Time: 30 minutes
Cooking Time: 10 minutes
Serving: 4

Ingredients:

- Boiled rice, one bowl
- Butter, one cup
- Eggs, two
- Crushed coconut, half cup
- All-purpose flour, one cup
- Coconut flour, one cup
- Water, as required
- Baking soda, one tablespoon
- Salt, a pinch
- Cornstarch, half cup

Instructions:

1. Take a large bowl and dry it well.
2. Add the sugar and baking soda.
3. Add the salt and cream.
4. Mix all the ingredients well.
5. Add the beaten eggs into the mixture.
6. Add the boiled rice into it.
7. Boil the whole mixture for fifteen minutes.
8. Cool it down in a large bowl.
9. Refrigerate it for fifty minutes.
10. Garnish the pudding with crushed coconut.
11. Your dish is ready to be served.

4.8 Vietnamese Apricot Tapioca Recipe

Preparation Time: 10 minutes
Cooking Time: 20 minutes
Serving: 4

Ingredients:

- Sliced apricot, one cup
- Baking powder, four teaspoon
- Coconut milk, one cup
- Baking soda, one teaspoon
- Eggs, two

- Brown sugar, one cup
- Tapioca starch, one tablespoon
- Salt, to taste

Instructions:
1. Take a large bowl and add the eggs into it.
2. Beat the eggs until they turn frothy.
3. Add the baking powder and coconut milk into it.
4. Add the brown sugar and beat the mixture for five minutes.
5. Add all the dried ingredients into a separate bowl.
6. Mix both dried and the wet ingredients thoroughly.
7. Cook the mixture.
8. Add the tapioca starch into the mixture and cook.
9. Put the apricot slices on cooked material.
10. Your dish is ready to be served.

4.9 Vietnamese Rice Balls Recipe

Preparation Time: 10 minutes
Cooking Time: 40 minutes
Serving: 4

Ingredients:

- Salted butter, one cup
- Rice flour, three and a half cup
- Black sesame seeds, one cup
- Yeast, one tablespoon
- Large eggs, two
- Kosher salt, half teaspoon
- Almond slices, one cup
- Vanilla extract, one teaspoon
- White sugar, half cup

Instructions:
1. Take a large bowl and add all the ingredients into it.
2. Mix everything well to form a semi solid mixture.
3. Add the formed mixture into a pipping bag.
4. Make small round balls on a baking dish and bake the balls.
5. Your dish is ready to be served.

4.10 Vietnamese Mung Bean Cake Recipe

Preparation Time: 30 minutes
Cooking Time: 25 minutes
Serving: 4

Ingredients:

- Mung beans, half cup
- Butter, half cup
- Sugar, a quarter cup
- Ground cardamom, a quarter teaspoon
- Flour, one cup
- Baking soda, a pinch
- Egg, one

Instructions:

1. Take a large bowl.
2. Make the cake batter by adding all the ingredients in the bowl.
3. Make the batter and pour it into a baking dish.
4. Make sure the baking dish is properly greased and lined with parchment papers.
5. Bake the cake.
6. Dish out when the cake is done.
7. Cut the cake into slices
8. The dish is ready to be served.

4.11 Vietnamese Ginger Syrup Milkshake Recipe

Preparation Time: 10 minutes
Cooking Time: 20 minutes
Serving: 4

Ingredients:

- Ginger syrup, two tablespoon
- Banana slices, one cup
- Plain yogurt, half cup
- Sugar, half cup

- Milk, half cup
- Coconut milk, half cup
- Ice cubes, as required

Instructions:
1. Take a blender and add the milk into it.
2. Add the banana slices into it.
3. Blend it for few minutes.
4. Add the plain yogurt and coconut milk into it.
5. Blend the milkshake well and add ginger syrup in it.
6. Your dish is ready to be served.

4.12 Vietnamese Coconut Ice Cream Recipe

Preparation Time: 10 minutes
Cooking Time: 20 minutes
Serving: 4

Ingredients:

- Crushed coconut, five tablespoon
- Whole milk, two cup
- Rock sugar, one cup
- Vanilla extract, one teaspoon

Instructions:

1. Take a bowl and add the milk into it.
2. Add the sugar as required.
3. Mix them thoroughly.
4. Add the coconut and vanilla extract in the mixture.
5. Refrigerate the mixture for one night.
6. Your dish is ready to be served.

4.13 Vietnamese Coconut Jello Recipe

Preparation Time: 40 minutes
Cooking Time: 10 minutes
Serving: 4

Ingredients:

- Fresh longans, one pound
- Coconut juice, one liter
- Agar powder, fifteen grams
- Rock sugar, two hundred grams
- Coconut syrup, two teaspoon
- Water, half liter
- Condensed milk, one cup

Instructions:

1. Peel the longans and remove seeds from them.

2. Grind the longans and set aside.
3. Take a bowl and add the rock sugar and jelly powder in it.
4. Add the coconut water into the bowl and mix well.
5. Heat the mixture so that all ingredients get dissolved.
6. Add the coconut syrup into the mixture.
7. Add the clear agar jelly in both bowls.
8. Add the condensed milk in it and mix well.
9. Add the grinded longans and mix well.
10. Your colored jelly is ready to be served.

4.14 Vietnamese Steamed Cake Recipe

Preparation Time: 20 minutes
Cooking Time: 20 minutes
Serving: 4

Ingredients:

- Baking soda, four teaspoon
- Coconut flakes, one and a half cup
- Baking soda, one teaspoon
- Buttermilk, two cups
- White sugar, one cup
- Water, two cups
- Tapioca flour, one cup
- Coconut cream, half cup

Instructions:
1. Take a large bowl and add the tapioca flour into it.
2. Add the white sugar into the mixture as required.
3. Add the baking soda and beat the mixture for five more minutes.
4. Add coconut flakes into it.
5. Add the coconut cream and water into the mixture.
6. Bake the cake batter in steam.
7. Your dish is ready to be served.

4.15 Vietnamese Wedding Cake Recipe

Preparation Time: 20 minutes
Cooking Time: 30 minutes
Serving: 2

Ingredients:

- Water, four cups
- Starch flour, one pound
- Sugar, one and a quarter cup
- Sugar syrup, a quarter cup
- Yellow mung beans, half cup
- Coconut flakes, half cup
- Vegetable oil, half cup
- Lemon extract, one teaspoon

Instructions:

1. Take a large bowl.
2. Add the wet ingredients into the bowl.
3. Mix all the ingredients well.
4. Add the dried ingredients into the bowl.
5. Mix everything well,
6. Add the cake batter into a greased baking dish.
7. Bake the cake for about thirty minutes.
8. Your dish is ready to be served.

Chapter 5: The World of Vietnamese Snack Recipes

Vietnamese snacks are famous all around the world. Following are some amazing Vietnamese snack recipes that are rich in healthy nutrients and you can easily make them with the detailed instructions list in each recipe:

5.1 Crispy Vietnamese Pork Rolls Recipe

Preparation Time: 30 minutes
Cooking Time: 25 minutes
Serving: 4

Ingredients:

- Bread rolls, as needed
- Pate, half cup
- Whole egg mayonnaise, two tablespoon
- Lebanese cucumber, one
- Roasted pork, one cup
- Red chili, one tablespoon
- Coriander leaves, five
- Onions, one
- Carrot, one
- White sugar, half cup
- Rice wine vinegar, half cup
- Salt, to taste
- Black pepper, to taste

Instructions:
1. Take a saucepan and add the sugar in it.
2. Add the vinegar, salt and pepper and cook it for five minutes.
3. Cook it until all sugar is dissolved.
4. Add the carrot and toss to coat.
5. You have prepared the pickled carrot.
6. Take the bread rolls and spread the pate over it.
7. Spread the mayonnaise over it evenly.
8. Add the pickled carrot, cucumber and pork on top of it.
9. Top with chili, coriander and onions and fold the rolls.
10. Fry the rolls until they become light brown in color.
11. Your dish is ready to be served.

5.2 Vietnamese Egg Rolls Recipe

Preparation Time: 40 minutes
Cooking Time: 30 minutes
Serving: 4

Ingredients:

- Egg roll wrappers, one package
- Noodles, half cup
- Whole egg mayonnaise, two tablespoon
- Lebanese cucumber, one
- Mushrooms, half cup
- Red chili, one tablespoon
- Coriander leaves, five
- Onions, one
- Carrot, one
- White sugar, half cup
- Rice wine vinegar, half cup
- Sea Salt, to taste
- Jicama, half cup

Instructions:
1. Take a saucepan and add the sugar in it.
2. Add the vinegar, salt and pepper and cook it for five minutes.
3. Cook it until all sugar is dissolved.
4. Add the carrot and toss to coat.
5. You have prepared the pickled carrot.
6. Take the egg roll wrappers and spread the noodles and mushrooms over it.
7. Spread the mayonnaise over it evenly.
8. Add the pickled carrot, cucumber and jicama on top of it.
9. Top with chili, coriander and onions and close the rolls.
10. Fry the rolls until they become light brown in color.
11. Your dish is ready to be served.

5.3 Vietnamese Squid Roll Recipe

Preparation Time: 30 minutes
Cooking Time: 20 minutes
Serving: 4

Ingredients:

- Chopped squid, half pound
- Spring roll wrappers, as needed
- Whole egg mayonnaise, two tablespoon
- Red chili, one tablespoon
- Coriander leaves, five
- Onions, one
- Carrot, one
- White sugar, half cup
- Rice wine vinegar, half cup
- Salt, to taste
- Garlic cloves, two
- Grated ginger, one tablespoon

Instructions:

1. Take a saucepan and add the sugar in it.
2. Add the vinegar, salt and pepper and cook it for five minutes.
3. Cook it until all sugar is dissolved.
4. Add the carrot and toss to coat.
5. You have prepared the pickled carrot.
6. Take the spring roll wrappers and spread the garlic paste and ginger over it.
7. Spread the mayonnaise over it evenly.
8. Add the pickled carrot, chopped squids and salt on top of it.
9. Top with chili, coriander and onions and close the rolls.
10. Fry the rolls until they become light brown in color.
11. Your dish is ready to be served.

5.4 Vietnamese Shrimp Wonton Recipe

Preparation Time: 30 minutes
Cooking Time: 25 minutes
Serving: 4

Ingredients:

- Wonton roll wrappers, one package
- Chopped shrimp, half pound
- Noodles, half cup
- Whole egg mayonnaise, two tablespoon
- Lebanese cucumber, one
- Mushrooms, half cup
- Red chili, one tablespoon
- Coriander leaves, five
- Onions, one
- Carrot, one
- White sugar, half cup
- Rice wine vinegar, half cup
- Sea Salt, to taste
- Pepper, to taste

Instructions:
1. Take a saucepan and add the sugar in it.
2. Add the vinegar, salt and pepper and cook it for five minutes.
3. Cook it until all sugar is dissolved.
4. Add the carrot and toss to coat.
5. You have prepared the pickled carrot.
6. Take the wonton roll wrappers and spread the noodles and mushrooms over it.
7. Spread the mayonnaise over it evenly.
8. Add the pickled carrot, cucumber and chopped shrimp on top of it.
9. Top with chili, coriander and onions and close the rolls.
10. Fry the rolls until they become light brown in color.
11. Your dish is ready to be served.

5.5 Vietnamese Rice Paper Salad Recipe

Preparation Time: 10 minutes
Cooking Time: 30 minutes
Serving: 2

Ingredients:

- Sheets of rice paper, as needed
- Date, one teaspoon
- Oil, one tablespoon
- Chopped green onions, half cup
- Mushrooms, as needed
- Maple syrup, one teaspoon
- Lime juice, two tablespoon
- Roasted peanuts, two tablespoon
- Cilantro, to sprinkle
- Soy sauce, one teaspoon
- Green mango, one
- Salt, to taste
- Black pepper, to taste

Instructions:

1. Cut the rice paper in desired shapes.
2. Add the rice papers in a bowl.
3. Add the date paste and mix well until rice paper is coated well.
4. Heat the oil in a skillet and add the chopped onions in it.
5. Cook it for two minutes.
6. Add the sliced mushrooms, soy sauce and cook it for few minutes.
7. Add the green mango, maple syrup, lime juice and roasted peanuts in the rice paper bowl.
8. Add the cooked material in bowl.
9. Your dish is ready to be served.

5.6 Vietnamese Pickled Bread Salad Recipe

Preparation Time: 10 minutes
Cooking Time: 30 minutes
Serving: 2

Ingredients:

- Pickled bread, as needed
- Oil, one tablespoon
- Chopped green onions, half cup
- Mushrooms, as needed
- Maple syrup, one teaspoon
- Lime juice, two tablespoon
- Roasted peanuts, two tablespoon
- Cilantro, to sprinkle
- Soy sauce, one teaspoon
- Green mango, one
- Salt, to taste

Instructions:
1. Take a large bowl and add the pickled bread slices into it.
2. Add the onions, mushrooms, maple syrup, lime juice and roasted peanuts in it.
3. Add the chopped green mango, soy sauce and salt into it.
4. Add the little oil and mix well to have homogeneous mixture.
5. Your dish is ready to be served.

5.7 Vietnamese Carrot and Cabbage Spring Rolls Recipe

Preparation Time: 10 minutes
Cooking Time: 30 minutes
Serving: 6

Ingredients:

- Chopped carrots, one cup
- Chopped cabbage, one cup
- Spring roll wrappers, as needed
- Whole egg mayonnaise, two tablespoon

- Red chili, one tablespoon
- Coriander leaves, five
- Onions, one
- Carrot, one
- White sugar, half cup
- Rice wine vinegar, half cup
- Salt, to taste
- Ginger, as required
- Garlic cloves, two

Instructions:

1. Take a saucepan and add the sugar in it.
2. Add the vinegar, salt and pepper and cook it for five minutes.
3. Cook it until all sugar is dissolved.
4. Add the carrot and toss to coat.
5. You have prepared the pickled carrot.
6. Take the spring roll wrappers and spread the garlic paste and ginger over it.
7. Spread the mayonnaise over it evenly.
8. Add the pickled carrot, chopped cabbage and salt on top of it.
9. Top with chili, coriander and onions and close the rolls.
10. Fry the rolls until they become light brown in color.
11. Your dish is ready to be served.

5.8 Vietnamese Tofu Baguettes Recipe

Preparation Time: 20 minutes
Cooking Time: 20 minutes
Serving: 4

Ingredients:

- Tofu, one package
- Baguette pieces, four
- Cilantro, to sprinkle
- Carrots, two
- Cucumber, one
- Daikon, one
- Sugar, one tablespoon
- Rice vinegar, half cup
- Salt, to taste

- Pepper, to taste
- Olive oil, one tablespoon

Instructions:
1. Take a jar and add the carrot, cucumber and daikon into it.
2. Add the white wine vinegar, rice vinegar and sugar in it.
3. Set aside it for an hour.
4. Drain the tofu and slice it.
5. Take a bowl and add the olive oil, lime juice, garlic, ginger and pepper.
6. Place the tofu on pan and pour the marinade over it.
7. Coat the tofu fully and cook the tofu well.
8. Assemble the baguette with mayo, tofu slices, pickled vegetables and cilantro.
9. Your dish is ready to be served.

5.9 Vietnamese Beef Tacos Recipe

Preparation Time: 30 minutes
Cooking Time: 30 minutes
Serving: 4

Ingredients:

- Garlic cloves, two
- Beef, half pound
- Lime, one
- Red onion, one
- Red bell pepper, one
- Lettuce, one
- Tamari, two tablespoon
- Sweet chili sauce, one tablespoon
- Whole wheat tortillas, eight
- Sugar, two tablespoon
- Salt, to taste
- Pepper, to taste
- Cilantro, to sprinkle

Instructions:
1. Take a large bowl and add the canola oil into it.
2. Add the sugar and salt as required.

3. Add the garlic powder and onion powder into it.
4. Add the red bell pepper and lime zest in the same bowl.
5. Mix them all thoroughly.
6. Then coat the beef into it and refrigerate it for thirty minutes.
7. Add the lettuce, tamari and sweet chili sauce.
8. Mix well and season with salt.
9. Cover it and refrigerate.
10. Wrap the tortillas in foil and bake for ten minutes.
11. Cook the beef for three to five minutes.
12. Divide the beef among tortillas, top with cilantro.
13. Your dish is ready to be served.

5.10 Vietnamese Carrot Tacos Recipe

Preparation Time: 30 minutes
Cooking Time: 30 minutes
Serving: 4

Ingredients:

- Carrots, two
- Garlic powder, one tablespoon
- Zest Lime, one
- Red onion, one
- Red bell pepper, one
- Lettuce, one
- Whole wheat tortillas, eight
- Sugar, two tablespoon
- Cilantro, to sprinkle
- Pepper, to taste
- Salt, half teaspoon

Instructions:
1. Take a large bowl and add the sugar in it.
2. Add the pepper and salt as required.
3. Add the garlic powder and onion powder into it.
4. Add the red bell pepper and lime zest in the same bowl.
5. Mix them all thoroughly.
6. Then coat the carrots into it.

7. Cover it and refrigerate.
8. Wrap the tortillas in foil and bake for ten minutes.
9. Cook the carrots for three to five minutes.
10. Divide the carrots among tortillas, top with cilantro.
11. Your dish is ready to be served.

Conclusion

For those hoping to explore diverse world cooking cuisines, Vietnamese food is an extraordinary option to begin with. It utilizes everything from tofu to meat and to shrimp, so there is something to fulfill for each taste at your table. Communal eating is a characteristic part of Vietnamese cooking. So, it is consistently a smart thought to serve the supper with an assortment of sauces, fresh spices, and sides to enhance any dining experience.

This book covers the Vietnamese cuisine, making it easy for you to prepare your favourite recipes in your kitchen without any stress. This cookbook incorporates 70 healthy plans that contain Vietnamese breakfast recipes, Vietnamese lunch and dinner recipes, Vietnamese snack recipes and Vietnamese dessert recipes that you can undoubtedly make at home very easily. So, start cooking today with this amazing and easy cookbook.

www.ingramcontent.com/pod-product-compliance
Lightning Source LLC
Chambersburg PA
CBHW080629030426
42336CB00018B/3127